Nutrition for Pregnancy

Expecting Mom's Guide to Eating Healthy During and After Pregnancy to Make Sure That the Pregnancy Goes off Without a Hitch and That the Baby Grows up Healthy and Strong

By Laura Nicol

© **Copyright 2019 - All rights reserved.**

The content contained within this book may not be reproduced, duplicated or transmitted without direct written permission from the author or the publisher.

Under no circumstances will any blame or legal responsibility be held against the publisher or author for any damages, reparation, or monetary loss due to the information contained within this book. Either directly or indirectly.

Legal Notice:

This book is copyright protected. This book is only for personal use. You cannot amend, distribute, sell, use, quote or paraphrase any part, or the content within this book, without the consent of the author or publisher.

Disclaimer Notice:

Please note the information contained within this document is for educational and entertainment purposes only. All effort has been executed to present accurate, up to date and reliable, complete information. No warranties of any kind are declared or implied. Readers acknowledge that the author is not engaging in the rendering of legal, financial, medical or professional advice. The content within this book has been derived from various sources. Please consult a licensed professional before attempting any techniques outlined in this book.

By reading this document, the reader agrees that under no

circumstances is the author responsible for any losses, direct or indirect, which are incurred as a result of the use of information contained within this document, including, but not limited to, —errors, omissions, or inaccuracies.

Contents

Introduction 1
Chapter 1: A to Zinc 5
Chapter 2: Calories 18
    Caloric Consumption During Pregnancy 18
    Caloric Intake During Nursing 21
Chapter 3: Healthy Vs. Unhealthy Calories 23
Chapter 4: Necessary Vitamins and Their Sources 31
Chapter 5: Just how much is Too Much? 34
Chapter 6: Mommy's No-No List. 39
Chapter 7: What if You Can't Eat a Regular Diet Plan? 45
Chapter 8: Food Intolerance and Allergies 47
Chapter 9: Veganism/Vegetarianism 53
Chapter 10: Dislikes 56
Chapter 11: Post-Partum Diet 59
Chapter 12: Exercise 67
Chapter 13: When NOT to Work out when Pregnant 71
    Post-Partum Exercise 71
Conclusion 73

Thank you for buying this book and I hope that you will find it useful. If you will want to share your thoughts on this book, you can do so by leaving a review on the Amazon page, it helps me out a lot.

Introduction

Kids grow up too quickly. Soon enough, you are going to be waving them good-bye as they begin going to college, crossing your fingers and wishing for the best. You are never going to have the chance to nurture them again that you do today when they're safely within you tucked away from the exterior world.

This will be the final time in your life when it's a breeze to get them to consume their veggies, so make the most of it! You will spend the following 18 years attempting to persuade them that spinach benefits them and that the slimy stuff on the carrot exterior is just pulp, yet today you're deciding when it pertains to what they eat.

Correct pregnancy nutrition is an essential factor in appropriate fetal development due to the fact that the fetus is incapable physically to provide for itself, nor could it show any noticeable indications of malnourishment in between month-to-month check-ups as a newborn can. That implies that for the following 9 months, it will be entirely up to you to make sure that you are appropriately eating for 2, taking in the nutrients and vitamins which will aid you give birth to a healthy, pleased baby while maintaining yourself healthy simultaneously.

Keep in mind that the baby is going to take what it requires long before those nutrients ever have the chance to go through your system. By not eating appropriately, you're not just damaging your child; you're hurting yourself too. That's why it's so essential that you ensure you obtain the nutrients and vitamins which you require for the next 9 months too. Mommy has to be healthy as well so as to keep up with her small bundle of joy in the coming months. Delivering is sufficiently tough on the body. You definitely do not wish to add malnutrition into the mix.

The issue that numerous ladies deal with when it comes to pregnancy nutrition is that they just do not understand. Why? Not due to the fact that they're dumb, or since they do not wish to do what's ideal for their child. It's due to the fact that a lot of pregnancy books, especially those which handle the ins and outs of nutrition for the following 9 months, are composed by medical professionals. Who better to take advice from regarding the development and growth of your infant than the medical professional that's made it their life's work?

The majority of moms aren't medical professionals, however, and that's where the problem can be found in. It's all fine to take a seat and look at a chart which demonstrates how much of every mineral you're expected to take in every day over the following 9 months, however, if you do not comprehend what you're reading and the impact it will have on your infant then it won't do you a great deal of good. You will spend a month, perhaps 2, taking a look at the labels on the back of your food. Then you will get fed up with it and go back to your old eating habits, thinking that you have actually always been healthy. You're taking your prenatal vitamins. What could fail?

During the coming parts, you'll discover a comprehensive breakdown of the nutrients you require to make sure that you deliver a healthy infant when the time arrives and fundamental guidelines for the trimester-by-trimester dietary modifications you will need to make, all written in regular English.

What's that mean? It means you do not need to head out and purchase a medical dictionary to comprehend what you're going to read! Even if you can't follow a regular "recommended" pregnancy diet plan (which has a tendency to become old after the initial trimester), you could still offer your small bundle of joy a great beginning of life.

Chapter 1: A to Zinc

If you have actually ever tried to go on any type of diet plan which entailed reading the information on the dietary labels of your food, you are all too acquainted with the truth that those small words and signs could begin to seem like Greek after a bit. If you're not a medical professional or a nutritional expert, you most likely have no idea about what Folic Acid or Vitamin B are, much less why they are necessary. The initial step to conquering pregnancy nutrition is comprehending what you're eating, just how much you ought to eat, why you're eating it, and how it will aid your baby.

A fast note. In the next part, you will see a number of mentions made about the unfavorable repercussions of overdosing on particular vitamins. You need to comprehend that this overdose really hardly ever happens due to the foods you consume. More frequently, it is due to the fact that mothers have actually picked to consume additional supplements in an attempt to "assist" their child, or they have forgotten to tell their doctor about other supplements and vitamins they take on a routine basis. Make certain when you go in for your prenatal appointments that your doctor understands precisely which medications, vitamins, and supplements (including herbal) you take, despite how irrelevant you might think them to be.

1. Vitamin A: Vitamin An assists with the development of baby's teeth and bones, along with their heart, eyes, ears, and immunity. Vitamin A shortage has actually been linked with vision issues, and that is why your mom always reminded you to eat your carrots when you were younger! Getting ample Vitamin A throughout pregnancy is going to additionally aid your body fix the damage brought on by giving birth.

Pregnant women ought to consume a minimum of 770 micrograms (or 2565 IU, as it is labeled on dietary labels) of Vitamin A daily, and that number nearly doubles when nursing to 1300 micrograms (4,330 IU). Understand, nevertheless, that Vitamin A overdosing could lead to liver toxicity and birth defects. Your maximum intake ought to be 3000 mcg (10,000 IU) daily.

Vitamin A could be discovered in carrots, liver, kale spinach collard greens, sweet potatoes, eggs, cantaloupe, peas and mangos.

2. Vitamin B6: Additionally referred to as Pyridoxine, Vitamin B6 aids with your baby's brain and nerve system development. It additionally aids Mom and baby establish brand-new red blood cells. Strangely enough, B6 has actually been recognize to aid relieve morning sickness in certain pregnant women.

Pregnant women ought to take in at least 1.9 mg daily of Vitamin B6. That amount increases a little when nursing to 2.0 mg daily.

Vitamin B6 could be discovered in fortified cereals, in addition to baked potatoes, bananas, chickpeas, watermelon, and chicken breast.

3. Vitamin B12: Vitamin B12 works with folic acid to assist both baby and Mom with generating healthy red blood cells, and it aids cultivate the nerve system and fetal brain. The body stores years' worth

of B12 away, so unless you are a vegan or experience pernicious anemia, the chance of a B12 shortage is really slim.

Pregnant women ought to take in a minimum of 2.6 mcg (104 IU) of B12 daily, nursing mothers 2.8 mcg (112 IU).

Vitamin B12 could be discovered in poultry, red meat, shellfish, fish, dairy foods and eggs. If you are a vegan, you are going to have the ability to discover B12 fortified tofu and soymilk. Other foods are fortified at the producer's discretion.

4. Vitamin C: Vitamin C aids the body to take in iron and develop a healthy immune system in both mom and child. It additionally holds the cells together, assisting the body to develop tissue. Considering that the daily recommended allowance of vitamin C is so simple to take in by consuming the appropriate foods, supplementation is hardly ever required.

Pregnant ladies ought to take in at least 80-85 mg of Vitamin C each day, nursing mothers at least 120 mg daily.

Vitamin C could be discovered in raspberries, citrus fruits, green beans, bell peppers, papaya, strawberries, broccoli, potatoes, and tomatoes.

5. Calcium: Calcium develops your baby's bones and assists its heart and brain. Calcium consumption increases considerably during pregnancy. Women with calcium shortage at any point in their lives are more probable to struggle with conditions like osteoporosis that directly impact the bones.

Pregnant ladies ought to consume at least 1200 mg of calcium daily, nursing moms 1000 mg daily.

Calcium could be discovered in dairy items, like cheese, milk, yogurt and, to a lesser degree, ice cream, in addition to fortified juices, cereal and butter, broccoli, spinach, sweet potatoes, okra, tofu, lentils, Chinese cabbage, broccoli and kale. It is additionally widely offered in supplement form.

6. Vitamin D: Vitamin D aids the body take in calcium, resulting in healthy bones for both mom and baby.

Females who are nursing or pregnant ought to take in at least 2000 IU of Vitamin D daily. Babies require more Vitamin D than adult babies, which means that your physician may recommend this. Do not worry. You have not done anything wrong! The formula is fortified with Vitamin D, so in case you are supplementing or bottle-feeding with formula, your baby is most likely getting ample amounts of this crucial nutrient.

Vitamin D is hardly ever discovered in ample amounts in common foods. It could, nevertheless, be discovered in milk (the majority of milk is fortified) along with eggs, fortified cereals, and fatty fish such as salmon, mackerel and catfish. Vitamin D is additionally discovered in sunlight, so women and kids found to have a moderate Vitamin D shortage might be told to spend more time in the sun.

7. Vitamin E: Vitamin E aids the baby's body to form and utilize its red blood cells and muscles. The absence of Vitamin E throughout pregnancy has actually been linked with pre-eclampsia (a condition resulting in exceedingly high blood pressure and fluid retention) and low birth weight. On the other hand, Vitamin E overdose has actually been tentatively linked with stillbirth in moms who "self-medicated" with supplements.

Pregnant women ought to take in at least 20 mg of Vitamin E daily, yet not more than 540 mg.

Vitamin E could be discovered naturally in wheat germ, vegetable oil, spinach, nuts, and fortified cereals and also in supplemental form. Natural Vitamin E is much better for your baby than artificial, so make certain to consume a great deal of Vitamin E abundant foods before you grab your supplement bottle.

8. Folic Acid: Additionally referred to as Vitamin B9 or Folate, Folic Acid is an essential part of your baby's development. The body utilizes Folic Acid for the DNA replication, tissue development and cell

growth. A Folic Acid shortage throughout pregnancy could result in neural tube problems like spina bifida (a condition in which the spine does not form entirely), anencephaly (brain underdevelopment) and encephalocele (a condition in which brain tissue protrudes out to the skin from an abnormal skull opening). All of these conditions happen throughout the initial 28 days of fetal growth, generally before Mom even understands she's pregnant, and that is why it is essential for women who might end up being or are attempting to conceive to get ample Folic Acid in their diet regularly.

Pregnant women ought to take in at least 0.6-0.8 mg of Folic Acid each day.

Folic Acid could be discovered in orange juice, oranges, strawberries, leafy veggies, beets, spinach, cauliflower, broccoli, pasta, peas, nuts, beans, and sunflower seeds, and also in fortified cereals and supplements.

9. Iron: Iron assists your body to form the additional blood that it will require to keep baby and you healthy, in addition to assisting to form the

placenta and develop the baby's cells. Women are seldom able to take in ample iron throughout their pregnancy through eating alone, so iron supplements, together with prenatal vitamins, are frequently prescribed.

Women who are pregnant ought to have at least 27 mg of iron daily, even though the Center for Disease Control recommends that all ladies take a supplement consisting of at least 30 mg. The additional iron seldom leads to side effects; nevertheless, overdosing on iron supplements could be extremely damaging for both your baby and you by resulting in iron accumulation in the cells.

Iron could be discovered in poultry and red meat, which are your ideal option, along with legumes, veggies, fortified cereals and certain grains.

10. Niacin: Additionally referred to as Vitamin B3, Niacin is accountable for supplying energy for your baby to develop in addition to constructing the placenta. It additionally aid to keep Mom's digestive system running normally.

Pregnant women ought to have an intake of at least 18 mg of Niacin daily.

Niacin could be discovered in foods which are high in protein, like meats, eggs, peanuts and fish, along with whole grains, bread, milk and fortified cereals.

11. Protein: Protein is the foundation of the body's cells, and as such, it is extremely crucial to the development and growth of each part of your baby's body throughout pregnancy. This is essential in the 2nd and 3rd trimester, when both mom and baby are growing the quickest.

Nursing and pregnant women ought to take in at least 70g of protein daily, and that is around 25g more than the ordinary women requires prior to pregnancy.

Protein could be discovered organically in poultry, beans, fish, red meats, eggs, shellfish, cheese, milk, yogurt and tofu. It is additionally available in supplements, protein bars and fortified cereal,.

12. Riboflavin: Additionally called Vitamin B2, Riboflavin aids the body create the energy it requires to develop your baby's bones, nerve system and muscles. Women with Riboflavin shortage might be at risk for preeclampsia, and when the baby is delivered, it is going to be susceptible to anemia, digestive issues, inadequate growth, and a reduced immunity, making it more susceptible to infection.

Pregnant women ought to consume at least 1.4 mg of Riboflavin each day, nursing moms 1.6 mg.

Riboflavin could be found in dairy items, whole grains, pork, red meat, fish, poultry, eggs and fortified cereals.

13. Thiamin: Additionally called Vitamin B1, thiamin aids build your baby's central nervous system and organs.

Nursing mothers and pregnant women ought to take in at least 1.4 mg of Thiamin daily. Nursing moms who are deficient in Thiamin are at risk for having babies with beriberi, an illness which might impact the baby's cardiovascular system (heart and lungs) or the nerve system.

Thiamin could be discovered in pork, whole-grain foods, wheat germ, fortified cereals, and eggs.

14. Zinc: Zinc is important for the development of your fetus since it helps in cellular division, the main process in the development of baby's small organs and tissues. It additionally aids the mother and baby to produce insulin and other enzymes.

Pregnant women ought to have an intake of at least 11-12 mg of Zinc daily.

Zinc could be discovered naturally in poultry, red meats, nuts, beans, oysters, grains, and dairy items, along with supplements and fortified cereals.

Keep in mind that the Recommended Daily Allowances are simply that-recommended. None of those numbers has been created on a case-by-case basis, so if your physician suggests something else for you, listen to what they have to state.

Chapter 2: Calories

Now that you're familiar with the different minerals and vitamins which you will want to have throughout pregnancy, let's discuss another subject which is near and dear to the female heart-calories. Because of society's devoted love affair with scrawny women, women who are less than thin have actually developed a sizable complex when it pertains to calories. They count them, they measure them, they burn them, and they factor them. They stay away from them anytime you can and are passionate buyers of anything with words "low" and "calorie" printed on them. In other words, ladies have actually made fighting versus calories their lifelong objective, committing themselves to it with a fervency which would equate to any religious zealot on the planet.

Caloric Consumption During Pregnancy

The initial thing you need to comprehend is that pregnancy is not when you should be counting calories. If you are on a diet plan that consists of significantly limiting your caloric intake, quit it. Immediately. For the following 9 months, you have permission to not suffer for beauty. Not just will limiting not lead to weight reduction (you're going to gain a bit as the baby grows whether you like it or not) it might possibly hurt your baby.

Not obtaining ample calories throughout pregnancy could result in the baby not having what it requires to develop correctly. Low birth weight is a typical issue, as is poor fetal growth. The baby might have any number of deficiency-associated birth defects. In other words, it is critically crucial that when you are pregnant, you eat enough. You could burn everything off after the baby is born, even though to be sincere, if you have time to stress over your weight, you are going to be dealing with brand-new motherhood far better than many!

The initial thing you wish to do is determine your pre-pregnancy Recommended Daily Caloric Intake. If you are a health enthusiast or have actually been surviving on a terminal diet plan, you might already understand this number. If you do not, you could go to one of the many websites to calculate it, or you can speak with your doctor.

For the initial 3 months of your pregnancy, you really do not have to take in any additional calories. Your pre-pregnancy calorie intake is going to be completely adequate for your baby's development and growth as long as you are not dieting. If you are dieting, stop! This is the amount of calories (approximately) that you wish to consume in a day.

As you enter into your 2nd and 3rd trimester, you ought to boost your day-to-day caloric intake by 300 calories. This is going to aid to make up for the growing rate of your baby's development. If your pre-pregnancy caloric intake was 1800 calories, you ought to take in 2100 calories a day. If it was 1400 calories, you ought to take in 1700 calories, etc. Once again, this is not the time to attempt and drop weight. Do not leave out these additional calories in favor of letting your body burn them. This is unhealthy for your baby or you, and in case you are breastfeeding you are going to swiftly work these calories back off.

The amount of calories you require throughout pregnancy will differ if you were not a healthy weight when you conceived. Ladies who were obese might be told to eat less calories to protect against extreme weight gain, and that would put additional strain on the lungs and heart and boost the probability of blood pressure-related issues throughout pregnancy. In this instance, this is a great time to diet, as long as you are following your physician's suggestions. The healthier you are, the healthier your baby will be.

On the other side of that coin, if you were underweight at the start of your pregnancy or have actually not gained what the physician considers to be a sufficient amount of weight since conceiving, you might be instructed to boost your caloric intake by more than 300. The baby has to be able to take ample calories away from your body to grow, and if you do not have any to spare either due to the fact that you aren't eating sufficiently or your body is burning all which you consume, they will suffer.

Caloric Intake During Nursing

Nursing moms usually require 500 calories more daily than their pre-pregnancy Recommended Daily Allowance. This takes into account the truth that the typical breastfeeding infant takes in 650 calories daily, and that is why breastfeeding moms normally drop weight far more swiftly than their bottle-feeding equivalents. The weight you put on during pregnancy is going to make up the difference. That's an immediate weight reduction of 150 calories each day simply by doing what comes naturally!

Those nursing twins who had little weight gain throughout pregnancy might consume more calories in a day since their bodies are not going to have enough additional weight to compensate. Once again, your baby is obtaining the calories it requires from your body. If you do not have ample calories to spare to produce an adequate quantity of breast milk, your baby is going to go hungry, pushing you to either increase your caloric consumption or start with supplementation.

Chapter 3: Healthy Vs. Unhealthy Calories

It is necessary to keep in mind at this time that no 2 calories are produced equal. There are 300 calories in a protein bar and a banana shake, and there are 300 calories in the typical cheesecake slice. Guess which one will be better for your child?

The challenging part of counting calories when you're pregnant is that you want to preserve a careful balance on numerous levels. Most importantly, you wish to make certain that you're consuming enough to provide your infant with what it requires. Secondly, you wish to make certain that the calories you are consuming are "good" calories, calories originating from foods which will supply your child with dietary benefits too.

On the other hand, you do not wish to consume excessive calories. If you do you are going to put on excessive weight, possibly placing you at risk for early labor, pre-eclampsia, diabetes and heart issues. You additionally do not wish to limit your food intake excessively. Pregnancy could result in certain quite extreme cravings, and overlooking these cravings could lead women to do certain outrageous things.

Unless you have one of the weight issues pointed out above, you are most likely better off considering your calorie intake guidelines to be simply that- guidelines. It won't harm you to go over from time to time and delight in a chocolate chip cookie or a piece of cheesecake. Simply do not do it frequently or too excessively. (Binging and consuming a half a gallon of chocolate ice cream one time won't harm you, even though it may make you ill. However, doing it daily might be an issue.).

Attempt not to count your "junky" calories as portion of your everyday required intake. This is going to aid you to keep on eating the needed number of "good" calories in a day, ensuring that your child is obtaining the nutrition which it requires. (That half-gallon of ice cream will account for around half of your everyday caloric intake, and suggests that half of the calories which your baby requires to grow today simply went down the drain.) It will additionally aid to keep you from doing it too frequently, because consistently eating 5 to 6 hundred calories over your suggested day-to-day intake will cause severe weight gain. The initial time you step on the doctor's scale and see you have actually gained 10 pounds in a month, the desire to binge flies out the window!

Not all "good" calories are made equal either. Here are certain fundamental guidelines for selecting calories which will meet your calorie requirements, your dietary requirements and your basic food desires. You have, without a doubt, at some time in your life, gone on a diet which has actually required you to restrict yourself to particular kinds of foods. The Adkins diet, for instance, significantly restricts your carbs, while the Sonoma Diet chops your dairy in half. What took place when you gave this diet plan a shot? Unless you are incredibly imaginative (or have an extraordinary amount of self-discipline), you most likely stayed with this diet plan for a short while, then tossed it to the wayside.

The secret to healthy eating during pregnancy is identical as eating healthy when you're not. You need to acknowledge which foods are ideal for your body and try to concentrate on them instead of their more appealing and less healthy equivalents. When you are selecting the foods you are going to eat during pregnancy, think about the following:

- Is it whole? Whole foods are those which are as near to their natural form as feasible instead of being processed. Fresh vegetables and fruits instead of canned, whole-grain bread instead of refined white and actual cheese fall into this classification. Whole foods are particularly great for pregnant ladies since the water and fiber included in them makes them much easier to digest. This not just helps keep you from being a lot more worn out than you already are since your body has a hard time digesting your food, it additionally aids you to reduce your odds of struggling with constipation.

- Is it a fruit or a veggie? Veggies and fruits , especially when fresh and/or green and leafy, are an important part of any pregnancy diet plan since a lot of essential vitamins could be found in them. Look beneath for a fast recap of the needed vitamins and the foods which supply them.

- Is it a good carb or a bad carb? You can not remove carbs from your diet plan completely during pregnancy. They supply both you and your child with the energy which you both require to be healthy and grow. What you could do is ensure that the carbs you eat benefit you. There are 2 main classes of carbs, complex and simple. Simple carbs are made from little sugar molecules which your body rapidly takes in. Instances of this are white bread, cakes, cookies, sweets and pasta. These are the carbs which you wish to stay away from since they are going to give you a fast sugar rush, and then leave you feeling cranky and tired.

The 2nd kind of carb is a complex carb. Complex carbohydrates consist of starches and fiber, like potatoes and whole grains. These carbohydrates require a bit longer to absorb, leaving you feeling fuller, longer and providing you the energy which lasts more than an hour or two. Naturally, even amongst the good carbs, there are some which will be better for you than others. If you are having difficulty eating because of morning sickness and struggling with fatigue as a result of hormonal swings, this is essential to understand!

So as to get the most punch from the foods you consume, you ought to concentrate on eating those which supply you with more energy, longer. That way when you can't consume as much as you did your baby won't suffer. Sweet potatoes and actual whole grain and whole wheat items are your ideal options, along with fruits like bananas and grapes. Remember that just because a package claims "whole wheat", "whole grain" or "multigrain," that does not always indicate that it is.

Yes, this is false advertising (kind of), yet it is essential to know. Food is just required to have a really little amount of whole grain so as to legitimately claim the title. It's not that there aren't whole grains in it, it's that it's not all whole grain. There are generally lots of refined and processed ingredients involved too.

- Are you eating the appropriate forms of protein? Just as carbs, there are good and so-so proteins. When you're searching for proteins which are going to provide you the most value, you ought to concentrate on eggs, lean meats, beans and beef. The less processed it is, the better it is for you. Does that imply you can't eat those chicken nuggets? Definitely not. Besides, when the sour and sweet sauce calls ... It does imply that you must not let processed meats end up as the dominant source of protein in your diet plan.

Is it organic? Organic foods are typically more pricey but are healthier than their counterparts. Organic foods, as specified by the Healthy Children Project, are those which are cultivated without "pesticides or artificial (or sewage-based) fertilizers for plant materials and antibiotics and hormones for animals. Genetic engineering and radiation are not allowed. Usage of renewable resources, in addition to the preservation of land and water, are emphasized."

If your budget plan will not stretch to include an all-organic diet (sadly, a few of those products came with a quite substantial shipping fee) try to concentrate on the foods listed by the government as the ideal to be purchased organically. These foods are more than probable to be high in pesticides or contaminated and consist of bell peppers, apples, cherries, celery, nectarines, grapes, pears, peaches, raspberries, potatoes, strawberries and spinach.

If you are worried about the foods you are consuming (and not purchasing organically) pineapples, peas, onions, papayas, kiwi, mangos, cauliflower, sweet corn, bananas, broccoli, asparagus and avocados have actually been judged the least likely to be contaminated or include high quantities of pesticides.

- What type of fat is it? Your body requires particular kinds of fat, however, trans fats (partly hydrogenated vegetable oil on the ingredients list) are hard for your body to handle and offers you no nutritional worth. Saturated fats are less healthy than unsaturated, are discovered in animal items like butter, and are ideally enjoyed in minimal amounts.

Chapter 4: Necessary Vitamins and Their Sources

VitaminFood Source

Vitamin A: Carrots, liver, kale, sweet potatoes, collard greens, spinach, eggs, cantaloupe, peas and mangos

Vitamin B6: Fortified cereals, baked potatoes, bananas, chickpeas, watermelon, and chicken breast

Vitamin B12: Poultry, red meat, shellfish, fish, dairy foods and eggs

Vitamin C: Citrus fruits, bell peppers, raspberries, strawberries, green beans, potatoes, papaya, tomatoes and broccoli

Calcium: Dairy products, fortified butter, fortified juices, and fortified cereals, broccoli, spinach, sweet potatoes, okra, tofu, lentils, kale, Chinese cabbage, and broccoli.

Vitamin D: Milk, eggs, fortified cereals, and fatty fish (salmon, mackerel and catfish).

Vitamin E: Vegetable oil, nuts, wheat germ, fortified cereal and spinach.

Folic Acid: Orange juice, oranges, leafy veggies, strawberries, beets, spinach, cauliflower, broccoli, pasta, peas, nuts, beans, and sunflower seeds.

Iron: Poultry and red meat, veggies, legumes, certain grains and fortified cereals.

Niacin (Vitamin B3): Meats, eggs, peanuts, fish, bread products, whole grains, milk and fortified cereals.

Protein: Poultry, beans, fish, red meat, eggs, shellfish, cheese, milk, yogurt, tofu, protein bars and fortified cereal.

Riboflavin (Vitamin B2): Whole grains, red meat, dairy products, poultry, fish, pork, eggs and fortified cereals.

Thiamin (Vitamin B1): Whole grains, fortified cereals, pork, eggs and wheat germ.

Zinc: Red meats, beans, poultry, grains, nuts, dairy products, oysters, and fortified cereals.

Chapter 5: Just how much is Too Much?

Now that you understand what you ought to be consuming, how do you tackle finding out just how much you ought to be consuming? The gold standard would be to walk around checking out small nutrition labels and keeping a little, continuous food journal in your pocket to ensure that you can monitor just how much of every nutrient you have actually taken in daily, but let's wake up and live in truth. Nobody has that much time on their hands. Due to the fact that you can't constantly monitor precisely where you're at with your day-to-day requirements, you will need to find out how to make some sweeping generalizations.

The most convenient way to do exactly that is to estimate just how much of every food group you will require every day, then choose foods from every group which you're particularly keen on, and that offers you with a variety of nutrients. An instance of a food group chart is demonstrated beneath:

Carbohydrates.

- Vegetables-4 servings regularly.
- Fruits-3 servings regularly.
- Whole grain foods-9 servings regularly.

Meat

- Milk, cheese or yogurt-3 to 4 servings daily
- Fish, poultry, meat or legumes-daily servings 3

Does that seem like more than you would be able to eat in a week, much less a day? Do not worry. A serving in this circumstance isn't the half a plate which your mom used to offer you. A ham sandwich with whole-grain bread is going to provide you with 2 servings of whole grains and a single meat serving. Include an apple to that, and you have actually just had one of your fruit servings too. A common meat serving is considered to be 4 to 6 ounces, around the size of a chicken breast which you would discover in a formal dining establishment. An eight-ounce glass of milk is going to provide you with a dairy serving.

A day's menu to fulfill all of your nutritional needs may look something such as this:

Breakfast

Banana.

2 cups of fortified cereal with milk (protein, whole grains and dairy).

Glass of orange juice.

Snack.

Apple.

Whole wheat English muffin.

Glass of milk.

Lunch.

6 oz baby carrots.

Ham sandwich made with whole-grain bread.

Glass of milk.

Snack.

Whole-grain bagel with organic cream cheese.

Glass of tomato juice.

Broccoli florets dipped in Ranch dressing.

Dinner.

Baked potato.

Trout fillet with lemon.

Whole-grain roll.

6 oz peas.

Glass of milk.

Snack.

2 pieces of whole-wheat toast with calcium-fortified butter.

Hot chocolate.

Chapter 6: Mommy's No-No List.

Just as there are particular foods which you ought to make sure to stock up on, so too exist foods which you ought to stay away from as if they would give you the plague in case you were to breathe in their general location if you were pregnant. Obviously, this list changes each year, so take the majority of these suggestions with a reservation!

If you're uncertain whether a food is safe for you to consume, or if you have actually heard mixed reports or have actually a worry based upon your private circumstances, contact your OB/GYN. Given that they are routinely required to take continual education classes and get regular updates from the research fields, they would be the most qualified to supply you with information relating particularly to your pregnancy.

Alcohol is initial on the list of No-No's for Mommies to Be, and for a good reason. The quantity of alcohol which is safe to drink in a day while pregnant has yet to be figured out, and the occurrence of known instances of birth defects because of alcohol consumption is on the increase. Based upon the March of Dimes, "alcohol is the most frequently recognized cause of damage to developing babies in the US and is the primary cause of avoidable mental retardation."

On a more private note, alcohol could additionally intensify a number of the typical pregnancy side effects like heartburn and nausea. It additionally uses up space in your stomach which could be filled with healthier things, such as juice or water. If you could abandon alcohol entirely throughout your pregnancy, that would be the ideal choice for your baby and you. Does that imply that a sip of your glass when you toast your cousin's wedding will leave your child scarred for life? No, most likely not. Utilize your good sense. While a sip of wine from time to time most likely will not harm your growing angel, a shot or two of tequila may not be as forgiving. Pregnancy is just 9 months long. Your child lasts a lifetime.

The other scare when it pertains to pregnancy eating has actually originated from a surprising source-fish. Long admired as the ideal protein source for pregnant ladies, it was recently uncovered that fish was additionally high in mercury, a condition brought on by the disposing of waste into the water. Mercury could lead to irreversible damage to a fetus's establishing nervous system. The debate regarding whether particular fish can be considered safe or not is still current, however, pregnant women are presently being urged to stay away from sharks, king mackerel, swordfish, bluefish, tilefish, striped bass, tuna steak, canned tuna and freshwater fish.

While extremely processed foods might not result in irreversible harm to your coming baby, they typically consist of ample preservatives to qualify them as highly questionable. Keep in mind, everything which claims to be sugar-free yet tastes sweet has some kind of sugar substitute. The question is, what are they replacing? Labels like "fat-free" and "caffeine free" ought to additionally be approached with care. Take the high road here and try to purchase whole, natural foods as frequently as you can. Take a look at the ingredient list on the label. The longer it is, the less probable it is to be healthy for your child.

If you have a tough time getting going in the morning without a cup of coffee, now will be the time to find out how. Caffeine hinders iron absorption, contributing to anemia in pregnant ladies who do not have enough to spare, robs the body of valuable calcium and intensifies heartburn all in one fell swoop. It additionally moves to your child through your breastmilk, which implies that if you like to drink coffee and you intend on breastfeeding, you could count on a great deal of late nights.

Even though you might switch to decaf, for the devoted coffee drinker, this is about the equivalent of taking a completely excellent cup of coffee and loading it 2/3 full of water. As a placebo, it's a bad replacement. Rather, attempt a cup of apple cider or hot chocolate in the morning. (Heating apple juice and including a bit of cinnamon works as well.) The hot beverage is going to strike a few of the "wake up" buttons that coffee sets off, and while you'll most likely feel the absence of caffeine for the initial week or two, you ought to discover that surviving the day becomes easier-and hey, pregnant ladies are expected to nap routinely anyhow!

Unpasteurized cheeses, fresh or soft cheeses like deli meats, Brie, undercooked eggs, hot dogs, fish, unpasteurized juices and rare to medium well meats are additionally being included at numerous intervals to the "no-no" list that OB/GYNs are giving out to their patients in an effort to halt the spread of pathogens like E.coli, Listeria and Salmonella, all of which are frequently present in raw or undercooked meats.

Listeria, the leading reason for meningitis in kids less than one-year-old, has the capability to cross the placenta and infect the infant. It could additionally result in miscarriage. Salmonella has actually been linked to stillbirth. Even if fetal death does not happen, dehydration from diarrhea and throwing up that accompany Salmonella infection is a severe risk. A serious E. coli infection could lead to dehydration along with potentially setting off untimely labor or miscarriage.

Identically, it is critically crucial that you clean your vegetables and fruits completely before you consume them, especially if you cultivate your own. You were most likely informed by your doctor that while you were pregnant, you should not deal with cat litter as a result of possible Toxoplasma infection, a parasite which resides in cat feces. Toxoplasma is additionally present in the soil, especially in locations where cats frequently wander and do their business outdoors. There is constantly a risk of Toxoplasma showing up in commercially processed foods, even though it is less frequent than in homegrown.

It is better to be safe than sorry when handling Toxoplasma. The parasite could cross the placenta, infecting the child and resulting in long term damage or stillbirth. There is a 15% possibility of the parasite infecting the child if exposure takes place in the initial trimester, 30% in the 2nd, and 60% in the 3rd.

Pathogenic infection of the establishing fetus could be possibly disastrous, especially when it is brought on by an invader that an adult immunity would have the ability to fight off with ease. It is far more desirable to put in the time to thoroughly ensure that your food is pathogen-free while pregnant than needing to live with the repercussions.

Chapter 7: What if You Can't Eat a Regular Diet Plan?

As kids are subjected to more foods at an earlier age, the occurrence of food intolerance and allergy is increasing. Add to this the issues of diabetes, vegetarianism and veganism, metabolic disorders and basic dislikes, and you could create a formula which equates to trouble for a pregnant lady. The question is, what do you do when you can't eat an ordinary pregnancy diet?

The response is, get imaginative! If you struggle with a digestive disorder or a diabetes, or you have a significant metabolic disorder like tyrosinemia or PKU (and these are just a couple from a lengthy list that are generally detected throughout early youth) you most likely have a pretty good grasp of how to handle your diet to supply the most nutrients at a time without overdoing it. To be safe, nevertheless, it would be a good idea to speak to your physician about which foods you can and can not have (and in what quantities you can have them) in the future months.

If you do not have a condition that needs particular, direct medical oversight and you just want to make some changes to the diet plan demonstrated earlier, you will discover that it will be much easier than you would assume (even though you will most likely be quite fed up with your core foods by the time you deliver!) With certain dietary replacements, nevertheless, you ought to still have the ability to preserve a healthy diet over the course of your pregnancy.

Chapter 8: Food Intolerance and Allergies

Food allergies, especially those to soy, milk, wheat and nuts, could be a significant problem when it pertains to preserving an effective diet plan. It's really difficult to get ample calcium when you can't consume one glass of milk or consume a milk product! The secret here is to speak with your physician about recommending some healthy alternatives. There are some, like a milk allergic reaction or a peanut allergy, that are simple to work around with chewable supplements and calcium-fortified juices and other protein sources.

If you have either one of these allergic reactions, you ought to be extremely cautious to maintain your food basically isolated, something that you are unquestionably already aware of. Numerous smoothies and "Meals in a Box" include these ingredients in some amount or another. The severity of your allergic reaction ought to be thought about when you're picking your foods, but if you experience anaphylaxis, you will wish to remain clear of them completely. Pick plain meats and fresh vegetables and fruits instead of casseroles and stews, and attempt to stay away from gravies if you can't see the ingredient list.

Sometimes allergies are going to be more extreme in pregnancy, so if you had a moderate response to particular foods before pregnancy, you ought to manage them carefully now. Keep in mind, pregnancy is just 9 months long. Your body ought to return to normal eventually, and you can return to your favored drinks and foods then. Up until then, it never ever hurts to be on the side of fear.

In case you are allergic to soy or wheat, you might have a tad more trouble, considering that a lot of the foods you will have to eat to get your servings of carbs will consist of these components. (Unless you, in fact, have a soy allergic reaction, you are most likely unaware of how frequently it's mixed in with numerous foods.) You will need to thoroughly read the labels on the foods you consume, looking for any of these words:

- Soy flour.

- Soy.

- Soy protein.

- Soy cheese.

- Textured veggie protein.

- Textured soy protein.

- Veggie protein.

- Tofu.

- Edamame.

- Yuba.

- Mono-diglyceride.

- Tempeh.

- Okara.

- Natto.

- Wheat.

- Soya, soja, soybean.

- Couscous.

- Bulgur.

- Farina.

- Enriched/white/whole wheat flour.

- Graham flour.

- Gluten.

- Semolina.

- Kamut.

- Wheat bran/germ.

- Triticale.

You'll discover that these are featured in numerous bread items, so it would be wise to obtain your carbs from other sources. The list of nutrient sources supplies you with some appropriate alternatives, so do not feel that you need to eat a specific food even if it's on your list. If you have preexisting health conditions, they need to be considered initially. Lots of women with a moderate milk allergic reaction or wheat allergy are going to intentionally deal with the side impacts in the interest of offering their babies with crucial nutrients. Pregnancy is unpleasant enough without adding to it by becoming ill!

If you are uncertain about what foods could be replaced in your diet plan without causing you to lose nutritional worth, make an appointment to talk with the nutritional expert at local health department or your doctor's office. They are specifically trained to assist individuals with dietary restrictions make the appropriate choices for their babies and themselves, and they are going to be happy to provide you their expert viewpoint and aid you in drawing up a diet plan that is going to work for you.

Food intolerance is one more frequent and yet often undiagnosed issue because the majority of people do not understand the distinction between an allergic reaction and intolerance. If they have a negative allergy test, they presume they're imagining things. That could not be further from reality.

Food allergic reactions are determined by your immunity. Your body basically identifies the inbound food as a foreign invader and launches something referred to as histamine from the cells. These histamines result in an allergy. Intolerance, meanwhile, has nothing to do with the immunity. When there is something which the body is not able to digest correctly, it rejects it, generally leading to digestive pain, gas, diarrhea, bloating and throwing up. Even though lactose is the most widely known digestive intolerance, it is in no way the only one. Veggies, red meat, soy, and particular fruits have actually been known to lead to it too.

You ought to stay away from foods you have an intolerance for, considering that diarrhea and potential for dehydration with frequent exposure could present you with some major side effects for both your baby and you. The ideal thing to do is to discover an appropriate replacement which will supply you with the needed nutrients without leaving you feeling as if you have to spend the remainder of the day in the restroom.

Chapter 9: Veganism/Vegetarianism

The newly found appeal of vegetarianism and veganism has actually made it simpler than ever to consume a healthy diet while you're expecting without jeopardizing your scruples. The majority of foods have a vegetarian or vegan replacement. Considering that you could still have fruits calcium-fortified juices (much of which have as much calcium as regular milk), soy milk and rice milk make terrific staples to your diet, and nuts and beans are exceptional iron and protein sources.

When you initially go in for a prenatal examination, you ought to inform your physician you're a vegan. They are going to most likely wish to go over your existing diet with you to ensure that you are consuming ample nutrients and recommend a supplement, in case they feel it's needed. In many cases, you are going to just have to include some foods to your diet plan to make up for the included nutritional demands of pregnancy. There are a couple of essential nutrients which aren't normally discovered in the vegan diet.

You might face some difficulty with your Vitamin B12 if you are a vegan and do not drink or eat dairy items, so it is critically vital that your physician is informed of your diet plan at your first prenatal examination. They might recommend a supplement for you or advise that you try to buy soy milk, tofu, yeasts and other foods which are specifically created for vegans and are strengthened with B12. A lot of fortified cereals additionally consist of some B12, so the following time you're at the shop, pick up your preferred brand of Lucky Charms and check the B12 content. You'll most likely be surprised pleasantly!

Vitamin D is one more vitamin which generally isn't discovered in the vegan diet but could be made up for by obtaining 20 to 30 minutes of direct sunshine a day. If your schedule maintains you indoor throughout the day, your physician might recommend a supplement; nevertheless, these ought to just be taken if prescribed. Excessive vitamins could be just as damaging as too few.

There are a number of terrific books out today on the subject of the vegan diet plan and pregnancy, and the majority of these include some awesome dishes. Put in the time to check out the diet and/or pregnancy area of your public library and book shop the following time you have an hour or two to spare and pick one up to assist you in assembling a diet plan which is going to to work for both you and your child.

Chapter 10: Dislikes

If you are a choosy eater, you might encounter difficulty when you're pregnant too, given that you're most likely going to get really exhausted, really rapidly of eating the identical foods or food groups repeatedly for the following 9 months. The majority of the time, you are going to have the ability to discover an appropriate replacement for the foods you do not like which are going to offer you with the nutrition you require for a healthy pregnancy.

The ideal thing you might do is go through the list of naturally discovered dietary sources and select 2 or 3 foods from every group which you can stand to eat. If you do not discover anything on the list in this book that works for you, then you can browse the web and do a bit of snooping around. You're certain to discover 3 foods somewhere out there that you can stand!

When you have your list, work on methods to spice things up! If you do not like pork and red meat, you'll most likely get bored of chicken eventually. Have a go at frying it up with a bit of lo-mein, putting it in a whole wheat pita with some raw spinach or slicing it up into a Caesar salad. Offer it with salsa, sour cream or cheese. Blend it in with your favorite pasta. The options are countless.

This would be a good time to purchase a cookbook. You'll most likely have the ability to discover one online or in your neighborhood book shop or library which focuses around your favorite protein sources. Because these are generally the main course in a meal, they are going to have a variety of choices for ways to prepare them, ingredients to mix in with them and side dishes to offer together with them. If you discover a big enough cookbook, you could most likely discover 10 or 12 recipes you like, then spin them through your weekly meal plan.

If you do not wish to spend the cash to purchase a cookbook, you could discover recipes for practically anything on the web-and it will not cost you a dime. You could even print them out to assemble your own cookbook. You'll most likely still wish to eat these meals after your pregnancy, and if you discover one you truly like it will drive you nuts if you do not print it out and you need to go back and search for it once again.

This is additionally a fantastic opportunity to attempt including some foreign foods to your diet plan, considering that many countries utilize the identical core ingredients in really different ways. Chinese, Latin, French and Italian foods are relatively simple to emulate regardless of what nation you happen to reside in because the foods you will require are universal and available nearly anywhere. This provides you with a terrific chance to broaden your culinary abilities and wow your buddies, family and colleagues.

Beware when you're cooking foods from nations which have a tendency to be heavy on the spices, because much of these might disturb your stomach and/or intensify heartburn. It is typically smart to cut the parts of those ingredients which are just utilized for spices by 1/3 to 1/2 while your stomach is more delicate. You could always include them back in later on, and it's a whole lot better than staying up during the night due to the fact that you do not feel well. You are going to do enough of that when the infant, in fact, gets here!

Chapter 11: Post-Partum Diet

No pregnancy and nutrition book would be complete without a fast blurb on what you should consume after having the baby. That so frequently gets overlooked!

Your post-partum diet plan will mainly be determined by whether or not you are nursing. We'll begin with the presumption that you're bottle-feeding because that comes with less guidelines! If you are bottle-feeding, then you do not have any uncommon nutritional requirements you need to fulfill. The diet plan you were on when you initially got pregnant is completely adequate, although until the delivery bleeding stops, you will wish to consume a bit more protein, fluids and iron than you would otherwise.

Obviously, if your diet prior to pregnancy wasn't all that healthy, to start with, then you might wish to make the most of the truth that you have actually generally spent the last 9 months adjusting your eating practices and give your diet a jump start. The initial thing you wish to do is forget about soda, sweets, cookies and junk food. These are all empty calories, and while the periodic chocolate fix will do marvels for your nerves when you aren't getting any sleep, it won't do a thing to assist you in dropping those pregnancy pounds.

Keep in mind, it took you 9 months to put that pregnancy weight on and it will take you 9 months to a year to drop it, in case you're Wonder Woman. It takes majority of women until their kid is between eighteen months and two years to lose the majority of their pregnancy weight, and in around 90% of the instances, an extra 5 or 10 pounds hang around simply to remind them that they delivered.

It is essential that you be ready for this, due to the fact that lots of women who fall short with losing all of their pregnancy weight in the initial 6 to 9 months with exercise and healthy diet plan turn to crash dieting rather, prompted forward by stars like Reese Witherspoon and Uma Thurman which seem to look beautiful and thin inside weeks of delivering. All of those stars who got their figures back within 3 or 4 months did it by hopping back into a stringent diet plan and workout routine long before you will be prepared (or able) to do so unless you have a baby-sitter and a personal trainer, so do not stress over it! The majority of folks will be too busy taking a look at a small bundle of joy in your stroller or your arms to focus on the additional weight you're carrying.

When you're trying to drop weight after delivering and you do not need to make up for the reality that you're nursing, you could cut your caloric intake down. Cutting 500 calories each day from your diet plan is going to enable you to lose a pound a week, a bit more if you up your workout routine too. When you're slicing those calories from your diet plan, make certain that you're doing it appropriately. You still have to take in your regular RDA of minerals and vitamins to recuperate effectively and get back into shape. You will not have the ability to do anything, including looking after your child, if you're malnourished or anemic.

As pointed out earlier, the first place you wish to begin cutting calories is in your sugars and fats. If you spent pregnancy peacefully delighting in the truth that for the first time folks, in fact, expected you to put on weight, you might have established an incurable craving for sweets by this point in time. If you find yourself continuously gravitating toward sweet drinks and fatty or sweet foods this is the moment to nip it in the bud. At this moment your body will be relatively accommodating about losing the weight you put on during carrying a baby. Make the most of that!

Following the fundamental guidelines set out by the Sonoma Diet is a fantastic method to tackle weaning yourself from junk foods and getting your dietary practices back on track for a lifetime of eating healthy. The Sonoma Diet basically places you through a 10 day "Boot Camp" which removes your fats, sugars, and high-calorie foods while still making sure that you consume enough of the nutrients you require to be both healthy and satiated. Even though you are going to be cutting your serving sizes, you are going to be consuming foods which fill you up quicker and maintain you filled up longer, so it's one diet plan you, in fact, will not need to suffer on!

The initial 10 days of the Sonoma Diet require that you avoid drinking or eating anything which does not fall under one of these classifications:

Water.

Black coffee.

Unsweetened tea with lemon (cold or hot).

Whole-grain bread (3 servings/day).

Fresh green veggies, like spinach, celery (which is incredibly excellent raw) or broccoli, which you could consume as much of as you desire.

Dairy (in tiny portions) 1 serving/day.

Low-fat sources of protein (lean meats, eggs, legumes) (3 servings/day).

At the end of the 10 days, you'll have the ability to see an obvious difference in your weight and you'll discover that the yearnings you had for potato chips, soda, and sweet stuff have actually started to subside. After that, you are going to be allowed to slip various kinds of veggies into your diet, like peas and carrots, along with an increased number of dairy portions and 2 to 3 portions a day of healthy fruits.

The Sonoma Diet is just a fast method to jump-start your weight loss and get you going with a healthy eating course. It is, in no way, the only way to go, so if you do not wish to spend the cash on the program, do not fret about it! Following the standards pointed out above for after the initial 10 days, attempting to cut sweets and beverages out of your diet plan and not allowing yourself to overindulge (eating despite the fact that you aren't actually hungry since everybody else is or since you do not wish to let it go to waste) is going to go far towards aiding you lose that pregnancy belly.

In case you are nursing, you will wish to be a bit more mindful of what you consume. Certain foods could enter your breast milk and impact your child, so you will wish to pick sensibly. Listed beneath are certain typical foods which lead to issues in breastfed children, so it would be a good idea to avoid them for a tad longer.

- Caffeine. You would not allow your child to drink coffee from a bottle, which is precisely what it will do when you drink a cup and after that breastfeed. While the periodic cup of Joe is not likely to harm anything, routinely giving your baby caffeine might lead to a budding young insomniac-the final thing you want when they're not sleeping during the night anyhow.

- Spicy foods frequently bleed through into your breast milk and lead to fussiness and gassiness in your child, especially if you did not eat them routinely throughout pregnancy.

- Alcohol. An infrequent drink of alcohol is fine (besides, you managed to wait for nine months) however, more than one drink could bleed through into breast milk. If you have had more than a drink, or intend to have more than one drink, wait 2 hours after finishing your last prior to nursing once again. Modest to heavy drinking which would lead to alcohol staying in your bloodstream for numerous hours is highly discouraged during nursing.

- Dairy. This will be a trial and error determination, as you definitely want to still obtain your RDA of calcium during nursing. If your baby seems picky or gassy after nursing when you have actually been eating high amounts of dairy, or if they show intolerance or allergy signs like diarrhea, hives, throwing up or eczema, try cutting down to see what takes place.

Aside from caffeine and alcohol, your diet plan isn't going to be all that restricted during nursing. If you see that your child is especially dissatisfied after feeding or more colicky than ordinary at the end of the night, make an effort to go back and consider what you ate that day. Was it anything you ate that they might have responded to prior?

Discovering whether a breastfed baby has a food intolerance or allergy is far more tough than with a bottle-fed baby, and it will necessitate a good amount of sleuthing on your end. For instance, say that you had the Kung Pao chicken for supper. It's now 2 in the morning and your baby is still crying. You keep in mind that this took place the last time that somebody brought Chinese home too. Removing Chinese food from your diet might relieve the signs, or you might need to try another thing. With a bit of experimentation, you ought to have the ability to get a relatively precise determination of the issue long before it ends up being a significant problem.

Chapter 12: Exercise

Because no genuinely healthy diet would be complete without a regular workout routine, we'll go on and wrap it up with this. The idea of working out when you're 9 months pregnant may appear dreadful at the moment, however, regular exercise has, in fact, been demonstrated to make both delivery and pregnancy go a lot smoother for both mom and child.

The days in which ladies were expected to take to their beds throughout their pregnancy are luckily long over, and if you worked out routinely before you conceived, you are going to take pleasure in having the ability to continue to do so up until delivering. The only difference between working out when you're pregnant and when you're not is that you want to be cautious not to overdo it. Women who take in too few calories while pregnant and exercise excessively have actually been demonstrated to stunt the development of their fetus, so do all things in moderation.

A great guideline to working out during pregnancy is that if you are too out of breath to talk during doing it you would most likely be better off placing it aside until after. This isn't the moment to begin training for your initial five-mile marathon, however, if you frequently work out twenty to thirty minutes a day, you ought to have the ability to carry on with your regular regimen. Your pre-pregnancy fitness will be the identifying factor in what you may and may not do while expecting.

One element you do want to think about is the effect of your exercise regimen. While high impact exercise throughout the initial 8 weeks (when you generally do not even know you're pregnant) hasn't been demonstrated to lead to issues, doing these exercises as you progress puts you at a greater risk of hurting yourself and, possibly, your child. As quickly as you recognize you are pregnant, you ought to think about switching to a strength-focused, low impact, training routine.

Yoga, pilates, walking and swimming are terrific for expectant moms, even though you ought to watch out for putting excessive strain on the abdominal muscle when doing Pilates. Dancing and step aerobics are additionally fantastic for aiding you remain fit if you can't stand the idea of quitting your energetic workout program. Strength training is going to aid you to develop the muscles in your neck, back, and legs, making carrying 20 pounds of baby around in your ninth month a lot easier.

Make an effort to stay away from anything which calls for balance as you roll into your 2nd and 3rd trimester because your center of mass will move and cause you to be more uncomfortable than you were formerly. Contact sports which might possibly lead to an abdominal injury, like soccer or basketball, ought to likewise be eliminated from the very start. Abdominal injury, even when unexpected, can lead to miscarriage at any point in the pregnancy. Your credibility for athletic prowess is going to be there up until you could properly get back on the court.

No matter what kind of exercise you select to take part in during pregnancy, you will wish to clear it with your doctor initially. This is specifically true if you have actually not regularly worked out formerly or you routinely take part in exhausting activities, like timed swimming or running, high impact aerobics. They might advise that you stay away from a few of the workouts you previously took pleasure in up until after you have actually given birth to help keep you and the child healthy and safe.

Be careful not to work out to the point of exhaustion and that you do not let yourself end up being dehydrated. Consume lots of liquids when you work out, and if the heat is harsh, stay within rather than getting ready for that trek you had in mind. Additionally, make an effort to stay away from working out either on an empty stomach or right after a meal. The drop in blood glucose you will get from not eating may cause you to end up being lightheaded and collapse while you are working out, and exercising on a full stomach when you have a baby pushing on it from the opposite side might make you nauseous.

Chapter 13: When NOT to Work out when Pregnant

In case you have a medical condition like pre-eclampsia or diabetes, you are at risk for pre-term labor, you have an incompetent cervix or you have actually experienced PERM (preterm rupture of the membranes, and that indicates that your water has actually already broken or you are leaking amniotic fluid) speak with your physician prior to beginning any type of workout regimen, even a moderate one. They might suggest that you spend time on bed rest to aid maintain your baby securely within you and growing for a bit longer, and working out in this instance might do more damage than good.

Post-Partum Exercise

The bright side is that when you have actually delivered, all bets are off. You could work out to your heart's content! The problem is that throughout the first 6 weeks to 3 months of your recovery period (longer if you have actually had a cesarean), your body will be recovering. Overdoing it at this phase is going to just drag this process out eve more.

Try to keep to the identical low-impact exercise program you took part in throughout your pregnancy up until you feel like you did before. In case anything feels uneasy or you find yourself become tired, stop and rest. "No pain, no gain" does not apply when you have actually just had a baby! You have the remainder of your life to work off those pregnancy pounds, so taking a couple of months to simply delight in being a mother and allow yourself to recover is completely acceptable.

Keep in mind that if you are nursing, you need to ensure you're taking in ample calories to offer your child while you're exercising. The final thing you want is for your baby to begin becoming malnourished, and breastfeeding burns an extraordinary amount of calories all by itself. You have actually already got a built-in, low-impact, extremely reliable weight loss system. Indulge in it!

Conclusion

Remaining healthy throughout pregnancy is not a tough proposition if you understand what you have to do. Women have actually been delivering for millennia, and the majority of them didn't have an anxious OB hovering across them every 2 to 4 weeks to guarantee all was moving along as it ought to. If you could follow the fundamental rules noted during this book and throw in a hefty dose of common sense, you are going to be well on your path to a delighted, healthy baby very soon.

I hope that you enjoyed reading through this book and that you have found it useful. If you want to share your thoughts on this book, you can do so by leaving a review on the Amazon page. Have a great rest of the day.

Printed in Great Britain
by Amazon